A CHANGE OF MIND

A CHANGE OF MIND

OF MIND

Looking at major depression

N. BIRD

A Change of Mind
First published by Summaculate, Manor Way,
Totnes, Devon TQ9 5HP
2009
summaculate@uk2.net

1 3 5 7 9 10 8 6 4 2

ISBN 978-0-9560962-0-3

Design by Andrew Crane
www.axisweb.org/artist/andrewcrane
in.spirit@virgin.net

Printed by Remous Limited, Milborne Port,
Dorset DT9 5EP
www.remous.com

CONTENTS

PREFACE

I am writing this because of all the times people asked me what went on. When I realised I wasn't communicating it I would just leave them with their versions of what they thought it might be. I want people to know more. I also think about it happening again to me and I want to clarify for myself what helped me to get through it.

1

BOIL WATER AND GET TOWELS

One thing you don't have to put up with when you have a broken arm is people telling you that having a broken arm is just as real as having a broken leg.

Yet sufferers of "major depression" are constantly being told that their condition is just as real as having a broken leg and that it wouldn't be useful to tell them to pull themselves together.

If it's said often enough perhaps onlookers will convince themselves. But maybe they won't, especially if they don't have an idea of what is broken or not working in the sufferers of "major depression".

For as long as the word depression appears in the name of the condition there will be confusion. We all know that pulling ourselves together is what is needed on some occasions with despondency and depression. It seems logical that anything called "major depression" is on the same continuum and requires a major effort of pulling yourself together.

Depression is a word that has been with us for hundreds of years to describe the discomfort and loss of motivation associated with lowered mood. It can be extremely unpleasant and it can interfere significantly with people's lives but it is unlike "major depression" in that when the sufferer's mood improves "major depression" does not start to lift whereas depression does.

"Major depression" is long term disorientation and agony of the mind which periodically immobilises the sufferer. It is a malfunction which can develop in optimistic people. During many stages of the condition the sufferers are not experiencing a low mood. It is not reversed by a change of mood or by alleviation of stressful circumstances.

Whilst experiencing all the various problems of "major depression", sufferers are likely at some stages, as an adjunct, to experience a low mood otherwise known as depression, and, to the outsider, it is the depression not the "major depression" that shows, because that is what is apparent and familiar.

It is almost impossible for a sufferer of "major depression" to conceive what is going on at the time, let alone communicate an account of an episode of "major depression". What becomes clearest to an observer are the symptoms of depression not the symptoms of "major depression". Depression is a part of almost everyone's life and so the signs are familiar and stand out. The signs of "major depression" are less visible and less familiar.

Not to identify "major depression" as separate from depression is therefore understandable.

But it would be helpful to make a distinction.

Consider the symptoms of painful contractions at the end of pregnancy. Though lower abdominal pains are part of almost everyone's life (usually something to do with the bowels) and the signs are familiar, it would be a mistake not to look further when they start nine months into a pregnancy. We need to boil water and get towels don't we, not just give comfort? We also need to do something more for "major depression".

We probably found it cumbersome after a few million years of dealing with pregnancies to keep calling contractions "major lower abdominal pains" so we gave them their own name. In the same way it is cumbersome to keep using the term "major depression" to describe what is actually a malignant change in the mind.

Let's be more accurate, stop confusing it with other depressive illnesses, and call it Malignant Mind Change Disorder, MMCD.

2

LET'S CALL
A SPADE A SPADE

GWENDOLEN: *I am glad to say that I
have never seen a spade. It is
obvious that our social spheres have
been widely different.*

The Importance of Being Ernest **Wilde**

It is difficult to identify a spade if you have never seen one,
more difficult if you have an inclination to avoid anything to
do with spades.

It is an understandable instinct to avoid anything to do with
MMCD and so it is not surprising that there is not a good
body of common knowledge.

But there is a very good reason to act counter-intuitively and
give some thought to the diagnosis and treatment of MMCD.
You cannot predict whether or not you may get it later in life
and if you get it, your recovery may pivot on whether or not
you knew in advance what to do about it.

Recognising MMCD in its early stages can be difficult. Its
beginnings are characterised by a significant disruption of
our thoughts and emotions. We are programmed to engage
our efforts to cope with such mental disruption and
discomfort in our daily lives by trying out selections from

many strategies we have employed at one time or another over our lifetimes for keeping ourselves mentally fit and able. If the situation becomes serious, we are likely to deny it is serious, because we know that confidence is normally half the battle of staying mentally well.

I wish we had a blood test for MMCD but we haven't.

Two people may feel dizzy and weak, one hasn't eaten enough and recovers after a hefty meal, the other has developed diabetes and needs to attend in a focused way over a long period of time in order to regulate his or her blood sugar levels.

In mental health just as with diabetes, we need to make a distinction between those who are experiencing distress from which they will recover without disastrous effects and those in whom there has begun a significant physiological malfunction.

My advice is that you decide in advance that you will go for help (see later) if ever the first three symptoms and one other from my numbered list below occur for a period of two weeks.

1. **You experience mental pain that is severe at some point every day.**

2. **Your sleep patterns changed abruptly and significantly. They remain changed every night/day.**

3. **Your eating patterns changed abruptly and significantly. They remain changed every night/day.**

4. You are often panicking.

5. You can't relax, find stillness or peace.

6. You urgently want not to exist any longer and/or have a great many thoughts about not existing any longer.

It may be that some sort of event has challenged your raison d'être (e.g. retirement/a significant blow to confidence or honour/moving from one country to another) or an event has been cataclysmic in some other way (e.g. a birth/death/ end or start of relationship/destitution/violence) or your biology has undergone significant change (e.g. onset of major illness/giving up or taking up heavy smoking/ drinking/drugs/giving birth). Even in these cases it would be sensible to take the appearance of the above symptoms as seriously as you would if they commenced out of the blue and not dismiss them simply because they can be associated with these triggers. These are serious symptoms. The sort of help to seek will be discussed later.

3

AN OUTLINE OF MY OWN EXPERIENCE OF MMCD

Sometimes people confuse MMCD with sadness - but it took me months of recovery from MMCD before I was able to feel this normal, healthy emotion again.

I have gathered some information about MMCD by reading and I have listened to several people talking about their experiences of living with someone who is suffering from MMCD. I have been told the bare bones of what happened to three people I know well, when they had MMCD. All the instances I have come across so far have individual traits but a startling degree of similarity in key characteristics.

I have had two episodes of MMCD, one in my early thirties and one in my mid forties. My two episodes were different from each other in some ways.

In the first episode I had a crisis period of about four months. I was too scared to take SSRIs (selective serotonin re-uptake inhibitors, often used as antidepressants). I took no medication during the first episode despite being strongly encouraged to by a psychiatrist: I thought it may increase my anxiety.

It took me about six months before I was sure that my sanity and my life were out of danger. I can describe here the analogies that I thought up soon afterwards but I can only remember snatches of this first episode of MMCD. When I was in crisis it was as if I was sinking in quicksand, slowly but surely. Despite doing my utmost to get out I was sinking bit by bit (for about four months).

After that I felt it was as if I had grabbed a large stick or branch and could stop myself from sinking any further if I could just continue to hold on. But I was still up to my neck.

Then from about six months onwards I felt as if I had found a solid foothold and could stand up. I was no longer being pulled down by heavy wet sand and I was no longer clinging on. I could look around and feel quite secure but I was not able to function properly, I couldn't step away.

By about nine months from the start, the analogy no longer felt relevant. I was out of the quicksand. But my view of myself was always in the context of surviving the MMCD. MMCD was like a huge mountain range that cast shadows over me for most of the time though I wasn't usually uncomfortable there. The presence of the mountain range just reminded me to make choices that would reduce the risk of recurrence of the illness. I would wake up every morning usually feeling ok and I'd think, "Oh, yes, I remember this. This is now my life and I've got to live it" but it didn't feel like my life. I felt as if I was taking on a role. For years my waking life didn't seem any more real than my dreams.

I was taking low paid jobs (I didn't regain enough

confidence to continue in my old profession). I was choosing a lifestyle in which I started to feel safe again. It was five years after the onset of the MMCD before I could say that I was glad I hadn't died. It wasn't that I was suicidal during those five years but I continued to think it would have been better for me if I had died before I had gone through that experience.

After that five year watershed (after which I was glad I hadn't died before the MMCD) I started to make my life my own again. I remember the return of bouts of happiness. I travelled, I took chances, I built a new career and though I still had significant problems with anxiety, at last I felt at home in my life.

Nine years later I was sitting in front of a doctor with a friend's hand going white inside my locked grip. MMCD had been brewing while I tried to carry on as normal and I had come to a standstill. This friend had taken me in and looked after me like a mother looks after an infant.

The time before (fourteen years previously) when I was in crisis I felt I was slowly being dragged to a point where I would be unable to go on. The second time I had MMCD the ending of my life was like a current need, not a future likelihood. The sort of agony I was in made it imperative that I end it straight away.

The analogy that I later thought fitted my second episode of MMCD was that I was like a beam carrying the weight of a roof and I wasn't strong enough. I was splitting and dropping towards the ground and the crushing from the weight above me was agony. The situation couldn't continue.

I was advised to take some SSRIs in my second episode of MMCD as in my first. This time I was offered a type that I was told are particularly helpful for people with anxiety. This persuaded me to take them. After a few weeks of increasing the dosages the intensity of the agony started to lessen.

Six months later I decided I wanted to carry on living and this time I was already glad I hadn't died earlier. I set up a survival lifestyle. I managed to continue my previous work (which I had developed over the last eight years and which was not stressful) on a reduced schedule rather than having to give up and find new work. I continued to cut off from the outside world before and after work every day and kept in touch with friends and family only by electronic means or a rare well-timed one-to-one meeting, in order to keep my life manageable.

Eighteen months from starting the medication I am still taking two thirds of the maximum recommended dose of the SSRI daily and (though not back to normal levels of energy) I manage well, I feel secure, I have times of happiness again (about four years earlier than I had in the first episode) and, most surprisingly of all, I am blissfully less anxious than I have been for the past fifteen years.

I now stand back as a matter of course from events I can't or don't want to alter. These days I am likely to find humour in the unknown. I am also likely to find humour in the absurdity of how my thoughts can occasionally turn to the contemplation of some detail of my life going disastrously wrong in the future without any reason.

4

THE NITTY GRITTY

I have recounted the timings of some of the events of my illnesses and recoveries. Now I am going to attempt to describe, in some depth, the experiences I had in the last eighteen months during my second episode of MMCD.

The beginning of the second episode was probably at the point I started to have many feelings of dread. Throughout my life these have been familiar to me, though they occurred infrequently. When I was very young I associated them with getting out of the bath and my stomach turning over and me feeling disconcerted. When I started to grow up I continued to have similar sensations from time to time and they started to remind me of feelings of homesickness. They were very vague physical sensations in my abdomen, accompanied by a feeling of all not being well (unaccountably). They passed within an hour or so and have never caused me any concern, they were just mildly unpleasant. I always thought everyone had them as a matter or course. People talked about butterflies in the stomach and stomach churning. I have since learned not to assume there is a universal similarity of such experiences.

In the run up to my second episode of MMCD I had to move house at very short notice and the dread homesickness sensations started from that point to occur more than usual. Although for some time I had been in an optimistic phase of my life, I started to suspect that my life, in fact, was a sad affair and the downs were greater than the ups. I felt bad. From a stance of optimism I had rapidly turned pessimistic.

I thought my change of outlook was a temporary response to my upheaval in having to move house. I was convinced I would overcome this blip by perseverance and I did. I did all the practical tasks that were necessary, I was very sensible. I paced myself and called on friends for practical help. I also talked to friends about my state of mind and got their support. I moved house and settled down again. The pessimism abated, normality was returning.

But when I took time off to give myself a treat or to relax, the homesickness sensations would arise out of nowhere, and they increased in severity to a pitch that became difficult. I recognised them as symptoms I had experienced in my first episode of MMCD. To all intents and purposes they were the same as the homesickness feelings but the physical sensations became aching, almost painful tension and lurching in the lower abdomen with a creeping sensation in my skin from my neck to my head, and the accompanying unease became an ominous feeling of impending doom. I denied to myself that I was having another episode of MMCD. After all, I'd got over my pessimism, I wasn't depressed and I was settled again. Life was looking good. The rest of the world seemed to me to be fine.

Now this is where those who haven't experienced anything like this may need to suspend their disbelief. I assure you that a normally rational person is capable of experiencing this. The ominous feelings of impending doom coming out of nowhere on a beautiful walk by the sea or in the middle of a quiet evening meal with a cherished friend, when all seemed to be right with the world, actually came to resemble feelings that you may expect would arise if you lost a child or if you saw your nearest and dearest being tortured. They were feelings of panic, horror and terror. I shall call these the lurching horrors. They came out of the blue, without an external cause, often without any sort of trigger, not even a thought.

There were a few weeks when I experienced these lurching horrors from time to time and then had several fine days without them when I would be optimistic, happy and normal.

But they got worse, happened more frequently and lasted longer. Then I started to wake at four in the morning and I would often already be in the middle of them when I woke.

I am usually a great sleeper. I would often get back to sleep but each time that I woke again I felt progressively worse.

I went from having a large appetite for food to being not the slightest bit hungry. Soon I felt nauseous at the smell, sight and later even at the thought of food. I sensibly stocked up on numerous small containers of simple foodstuffs for myself and made sure I ate by the clock, eating little and often, but I often gagged when swallowing.

I became thirstier than I thought it was possible to be and carried a big bottle of water with me wherever I went. I counted that I was drinking twelve to fifteen pints of water every day and still had a dry mouth and an impulse to keep drinking. In fact I felt dehydrated.

For several years previously I had practised mindfulness meditation every morning, but now I found sitting in silence, in order to let thoughts and feelings flow through me, without my engaging with them, became a task I was constantly failing at, which now exacerbated my problems. So I started listening to tapes for deep muscle relaxation. Also many times each day I would concentrate as hard as possible on noticing my breathing. I was continuing to wake at four in the morning and found it less and less easy to get back to sleep.

I wanted no sexual contact and it was an intense relief when I broke off relations with my sexual partner.

5

IT WORSENS

At some point during the weeks when all this was happening, a change took place. I was no longer feeling awful sensations through my normal senses. When I experienced the lurching horrors my senses themselves were changed. There was a new dimension opening up to me. A new dimension where it seemed that I was no longer experiencing terror but that the terror of the world and I merged in some way. The sense I had of my own independent existence changed. I no longer had the same human identity. I was becoming a blur.

Once the illness had set in, whether or not I was experiencing the lurching horrors, my mind had undergone a change such that mundane procedures of thinking and feeling were malfunctioning. Quite separate from the nauseous feelings associated with food, I also had a sort of seasickness of the thinking and feeling processes. It was like seasickness in the sense that I was unable to concentrate or feel things normally. To all intents and purposes my mind was affected by the force of another motion and no longer my own motion and it was uncomfortable and disorientating. It wasn't that other objects seemed to be moving around me it was that I was all at sea internally.

Also my physical, muscular strength was often sapped as if I had the incapacitation of the sort of flu that keeps you in bed without an ounce of energy (but I didn't have a headache, a cough or a fever).

Routines were essential. I didn't ask myself when I would like to eat or what I would like to eat. My willpower led me just to dip the spoon into what I had put by the bed, as soon as I woke up, without question. I put out the same things (rice pudding or yoghurt in little tubs, dried fruit and nuts, bananas) on a sort of rota and I ate them at regular intervals. I thought regular eating might make the illness go away.

Coming round in the mornings was often such a terrible experience I didn't think the body could keep itself alive for long when it felt so bad. I thought it would just expire but it didn't.

Being awake and conscious felt dangerous.

In the mornings I could not make my body do tasks normally. Occasionally I would crawl rather than walk, pausing to lie my face flat on the floor.

I started to make involuntary grunting noises, like a prize fighter, to help me in the gargantuan tasks of moving my limbs and keeping my feelings from taking me over. I sat heavily on the edge of furniture pressing it into my flesh, it seemed to channel the tension away.

I learned to prepare food and clothing and to wash myself in the evenings instead of in the mornings because, at some point during most evenings I could navigate (as if sleepwalking) my way round those chores but in the mornings each effort seemed to break me a bit more and leave me a bit more diminished.

More than anything, I wanted the anguish to stop.

In the forefront of my mind the knowledge that if I was dead I would not be in this pain, took up residence. What I feared most was staying alive in this state. If only I could stop existing without anyone minding. My willpower dictated I had to do everything I could to recover and at the same time I had an aim not to exist any more.

6

ROCK BOTTOM

Pitched past pitch of grief

No Worst There Is None **Hopkins**

There are two aspects of MMCD that are still vivid in my memory.

The first aspect is that whenever I thought I had reached rock bottom I found it was a false bottom which was cracking under me. A different horror would appear just when I thought things could not get any worse.

The second aspect that I remember is having a respite from the illness. I felt intense relief that I would be safe at last. I seemed to be able to think clearly and feel normally. Relief flowed through me. All was going to be well. When ill, I couldn't feel emotions normally but in the respite I could feel (with my normal capacity to feel pleasant emotions) that being well was wonderful. Then, as suddenly as it had come, the respite ended after a few hours, I was taken captive and I set about the task of managing to endure the illness again hampered by the agony of the mind, explosive thoughts and not being able to feel emotions normally.

The relief and relapses happened several times. Each time I had a respite the relief was phenomenally powerful. I told people I loved them and thanked people for their help. I remembered what it felt like to be normal again. It is difficult to convey what effect it had on me when the respites suddenly ended. The juxtaposition of despair at these disappointments after the surge of relief was the most hideous and destabilising part of my condition.

I lost trust in the ability I thought I had, of assessing what was going on. I was taught by my experience of MMCD not to trust my own observations.

I was also taught by my experience of MMCD not to trust my hopes. When I had the most evidence to build them up, they were dashed.

7

NO INNOCENT DREAMS

After a while I could no longer remember my dreams except for the odd atmosphere of foreboding or occasional vague ideas such as that I had murdered someone.

I didn't cry with sadness but often I could not staunch silent flows of tears when I found it difficult trying to speak. I woke up crying sometimes.

I was often incapacitated from doing any activity that wasn't deeply ingrained in me as my necessary routine (such as clothing myself and eating). Sitting in the sun was once a much loved means of relaxation which, it would appear, wouldn't require exertion on my part. But spring sunshine and a whole summer was lost to sleep in a curtained room. Though I continued to know I had once loved being in the sun, now it was inexplicably impossible. There wasn't any particular aspect of it that was difficult. I had the perfect space for it and plenty of time. When I finally did manage to go out in the sun, when I was recovering, I was bewildered and I wasn't enjoying it. I was finding it difficult and yet all the elements of it that I used to enjoy were there.

I had stopped reading. Not only could I not keep up

concentration on what the words meant but it was too tiring to try to contain the feelings inspired by the ideas and the associations evoked.

Similarly for about nine months, hearing music of any sort churned up my emotions to screaming point so I avoided music completely.

I soon learned not to try listening to radio or television broadcasts, even cheerful ones. They pumped out too much for me to handle. My ability to think wasn't up to the trials inflicted by trying to comprehend and process unpredictable information. My emotions, stimulated while listening, spiralled and shredded my endurance into tatters. I couldn't, however, countenance any silence. To be left without distraction from my thoughts and feelings was impossible. From the moment I woke to the moment I slept, I played tapes of spoken books that were simple and extremely familiar to me. Of all the tapes of readings I knew, there were only half a dozen that I could rely on to be bland enough not to be upsetting. I dreaded the end of each tape just in case when I turned it over, something had gone wrong with the player, or the tape had got chewed up and I wouldn't be able to continue to play it. I bought spare tape players and had them and earphones at each place I might ever have to be (I also had a spare in my car just in case).

I had a large collection of films on video and dvd. I selected out ones which I thought would be undemanding and with which I was very familiar. I would sometimes start watching one of these innocuous "feel good" films for a few minutes then reject it for being too disturbing. I would sometimes repeat this a dozen times before I could settle on one that would do. When I had chosen one and it continued to be ok I would often find that half way through it I was distracted out of the lurching horrors or I might have fallen asleep.

When I was taking tranquillisers I took to sleeping for an average of three to four hours at a time. I fitted at least three sleep sessions into each twenty four hours.

Minor paranoiac thoughts reared their head. When I was in public places I thought someone might be scrutinising my actions on CCTV to see how I was taking the illness. I thought my neighbours might be looking in my windows a bit too much. There were some old security cameras in my new house that had been disconnected but I covered them all up because I thought someone might be trying surreptitiously to film me (somehow). I recognised the unlikeliness. The fact that I had the thoughts surprised me a bit.

Obsessive and compulsive behaviours increased. I counted things a lot, my steps, my breaths in and out. I became very concerned that I could not clean my living area adequately. My ideas of what constituted cleanliness became more exacting, I felt out of control of the dirt that I imagined had built up. I had insufficient energy to do much about it.

But some obsessive and compulsive behaviours were beneficial. I used them to help me with maintaining my routine and helping me in not questioning but just repeating actions like food preparation and washing myself. I repeatedly checked, by counting to six, that I had my wallet, bank card, phone, diary, address book and keys to ensure I wouldn't mislay any of them and wouldn't keep wondering if I had mislaid any of them. List-making took away the pressures of trying to remember mundane details.

Questions about the future, for instance, "What time are you going out?" upset me surprisingly badly. I couldn't comprehend any longer how the passage of time worked and how I featured in it. My thought processes were not up to hypothesis. I didn't know what information I needed in order to work it out. I didn't want to speculate. I could tell you about something I had done, but not about the timing of something that I was going to do.

Certain smells and noises caused me problems. I remember on several occasions, being thrust, by smells of deep fat frying and by loud traffic noises in the street, into incapacitating mental pain.

Over time the lurching sensations developed into slow, deep, thudding pulses in the lower abdomen and there was such tension there that I found I often pressed really hard onto that area.

What I was suffering was not primarily a lowered mood.

I had too much information in my brain to process. It was as if, when I started to sweep the floor, more dust and rubbish appeared around the broom with every sweep. There was a deluge of endless debris the more I swept it and no longer any floor beneath it.

My efforts to think and feel normally were being ineffectual. It was as if my eyesight had rapidly deteriorated and I couldn't focus however much I tried. It was as if the lenses in my eyes would not respond to my efforts to modify them.

I couldn't rely on being able to organise my thoughts or regulate my feelings. Each effort was as if I was trying to fasten a window open and I couldn't get the catch to hold after numerous attempts. I kept trying. It was not just my intellect and thoughts that were affected, the mechanisms by which I managed my emotions weren't working. I could no longer rely on being able to move on from a feeling, as it could stick with me and amplify. It was rather like inadvertently or against my will recalling lots of songs with great accuracy when not actually hearing them and then not being able to get rid of them afterwards. In fact employing more tactics to dislodge the tunes seemed to recall more verses and then make them louder.

When I was trying to have a conversation it was like trying to drive a car in a gale on an exposed bridge when the steering is being buffeted. It took a lot of energy to keep control. It was a long time to the end of a sentence. I could do small talk but real conversations face to face and on the telephone were too much for me most of the time. I found text messages and e-mails very useful for the duration of the illness.

In my experience of MMCD an idea would fracture like in a kaleidoscope into a thousand painful feelings and scary perspectives however much I disbelieved those thousand.

Being approached by a friend unexpectedly, was terrifying. I was not good with surprises and the more heightened were the emotions that would normally be associated with an event (whether they would normally be pleasant or unpleasant) the worse the experience would be for me.

Symptoms that people often have when they are tired or overwhelmed were familiar to me. I would stand, unable to focus on goods in a supermarket, without knowing what information I needed in order to take something from the shelf. This was a time when unquestioned, simple routine helped. I got used to buying a predetermined number of a few different items from the same list.

Waiting for an unknown length of time was not dissimilar to the prospect of awaiting a bomb blast so, whenever I could, I cut out activities that required me to wait.

I found that feelings of dread increased at changes of activity. Changes of scene were difficult for me. Even if I was going back to the safety of my bed, the transition itself increased my difficulties. It was a bit like the dread at the ending of the tapes I played.

I didn't know what effect I was having on other people or how I came across, though I knew I once would have had an idea. I found that asking friends to give me feedback about this was helpful.

A glance from one person would often suggest to me several different unpleasant interpretations and scenarios and, though I knew that none of them had to be true, the prospects of some of the interpretations were very upsetting. It was like a normal malfunctioning of social skills amplified. Having a friend with me when I had to meet someone, helped me not only in recalling what had been said but also helped me see whether my assumptions and interpretations of nasty glances, tones of voice and body language for example were backed up by reliable evidence or not.

I was trying not to think or feel things. I was trying to want to survive and when that failed I was trying to fight MMCD until the very end. Throughout both episodes of MMCD I knew I had an indomitable willpower. I kept on mustering it and I could sense its strength but again and again by some inexplicable means my willpower didn't achieve the desired results. My willpower didn't flag and I knew the willpower was strong for the duration of the illness but it kept slipping out of gear and when it did I could only freewheel.

I often felt I couldn't carry on but I always did carry on.

8

CROSSED WIRES

It may be helpful, in trying to envisage what goes wrong in those suffering from MMCD, to compare the experiences of those who are depressed with those who have MMCD, in terms of the effects that certain thoughts have on them.

In order to understand this further it is worth contemplating your own personal list of thoughts which encourage you during your everyday life when you are well. I have drawn up a generalised list to prompt you to think of some of your own thoughts that can make you feel better from day to day.

being useful
buying things you really want
chatting
cuddling
cup of tea
delicious food
doing ok
drink
driving fast
dvd
eating chocolate
enjoying the look of your house
feeling quite proud you did that
feeling the sun on your skin
film

finding something in common with someone
finishing that job
garden
getting away
getting some money
going home
going out with a group of friends
having a break
holiday planning
hugging
impressing someone
kissing
knowing work will be over soon
knowing you do that well
laughing
lazy morning with papers
learning
listening to music
looking after someone
looking at your car and knowing that it is yours
looking good
lovely bath
lunch
magazine
making that person smile (they look much happier after they see you)
moaning to someone who sympathises
more information
phone call
pleasing someone
reading a book you're into
relaxing
seeing children happy
seeing how tidy it is now

seeing that person face to face
seeing that person who thinks you're ok
sex
sharing a joke
shower
showing that person you were right
sitting down to rest
sleeping
snack
something beautiful
something funny
sports
sunset
talking to that friend
team spirit
that person fancies me
that site on the internet
training to do more
watching a tv programme
watching sport
wearing favourite clothes
working well

Now imagine that every thought that flits through your mind about things you once looked forward to, and all thoughts that could encourage you, leave you feeling nothing at all. There is a lack of looking forward to the smallest or largest thing. Little or no expectation of success, reward or pleasure in the present or in the future even in the smallest detail. This is often the experience of those who are depressed. In addition to this absence of uplifting feelings associated with previously encouraging thoughts, a depressed person may find that their thoughts are predominantly particularly negative and evoke anguish.

Anguish associated with negative thoughts is also experienced by those with MMCD. In addition, the experience of someone with MMCD is that the thoughts that were once uplifting now do not bring an absence of feeling but instead an inexplicable shock of discomfort or distress. Instead of reassurance and pleasurable reward in the minor details of everyday life there is an electric fence-like setback at even just the vaguest prospect of something pleasurable. Somehow the wires get crossed.

For me, when a little pleasure or excitement started stirring inside me, my body translated it into discomfort or panic.

Evoking encouraging thoughts in someone with MMCD will not have positive benefits and could worsen the situation.

9

THEN THE JUDGEMENTS I MADE

When I was not ill I could let judgements pass through my mind. I could conceive of them as thoughts that I didn't have to give credence to, and, as a consequence, I could remain unaffected by them. When I had been ill for several weeks, judgements stayed with me and they affected me in spite of all my efforts. I was as incapable of regulating such thoughts as someone suffering from Parkinson's tremors can be unable to stop making movements.

I was plagued by these particular judgements:

I am going mad.

I am being punished.

I had too much fun during the rest of my life and I'm paying for it from now onwards.

I can't carry on.

I will lose the ability to earn a living.

I will lose all my friends.

I won't ever be the sort of person who can be called on to help anyone. I can't be reliable ever again.

It gets worse and worse.

There is no end to this.

I have failed and its final. My life is irretrievable. I am a no hoper.

It's all my fault.

If this condition could ever be halted I will be mentally damaged beyond repair.

Thoughts arose from feelings like vapour rising from a kettle and then, just as suddenly, worse feelings would arise from thoughts.

If a nightmare is the mind experiencing horror and terror which spirals out of control, then I was trapped in a nightmare.

10

ALLEVIATION

I've seen film of an Amazonian hunter piercing his nose with a stick without flinching. After months of the sort of mental pain I experienced, I had become a bit like that nose piercer. But being like this didn't heal me, it just meant I could endure mental pain without fighting against the pain.

Before experiencing MMCD when my mental faculties were not disabled I could successfully employ cognitive behavioural techniques and other methods to be at peace with my thoughts and emotions but when I was ill, efforts to do so actually exacerbated my problems. I found my confusion increased when I tried simply to notice my thoughts and feelings and let them go. I couldn't do it. This is what the illness incapacitated me from doing. The best I could do was distraction.

When I have a coughing reflex I can swallow hard and breathe hard and sometimes avoid coughing if I concentrate enough. I wonder if there are similar ways, when we are out of our minds with horror, or are unable to think coherently, that we could train ourselves to halt MMCD by our own efforts.

I know that when I had MMCD I didn't find the answers though I was preoccupied with searching for ways to alleviate symptoms and cope with them. Each day brought a new set of observations of what I thought helped.

"It's better now that I am eating something just before I sleep/ now that I don't eat any chocolate/ don't drink any caffeine at all/ when I've eaten dairy fats/ when I set the alarm clock to go off in three hours/ when I don't set my alarm clock at all/ when I don't have any schedule/ now that I have a set schedule.....it goes away when I hold my breath and keep holding it/ when I gulp down hot drinks/ when I press this part, that part....."

11

ON VIEW

I don't really know what showed and what didn't show of what was going on inside me.

I know that soon after my first episode several people said they hadn't realised anything was wrong at the time. The second episode was different. When I started to get better I had quite a lot of unsolicited questions about my health from people I hadn't talked about it to, they said I had looked ill and that my face had changed.

I know I had stuttered a bit and my voice hadn't flowed easily. I had also found it hard to remember vocabulary. But I don't know how noticeable that was.

During both episodes of MMCD I lost approximately a tenth of my body weight in the first couple of months.

Not a lot of external evidence really.

A confidante of mine, during one of the worst times in my second episode of MMCD, introduced me to her grandchildren. She said how good it was to see me feeling better. I explained I wasn't feeling any better. She then asked why I was smiling with the children and all I could think was that I thought that was what they expected.

It didn't reflect how I felt.

I think it is important to realise that, as sociable beings, we sometimes go onto an automatic mode of behaving and we reflect what is positive around us regardless of what is going on inside us.

Well considered messages may sometimes also be misleading. I scribbled on my calendar one day that my condition was particularly dreadful. That evening I sent e-mails to seven people saying "Will write soon, I'm ok". I think I was having one of my worst days and had chosen to write "Ok" to reflect that I was managing the extra difficulties. But my words didn't express that detail and may have been interpreted as an indication that I was quite well again.

12

HOPE
MAY NOT HELP

The illness progressed even though my circumstances were improving when I resettled in a new house. It had a life of its own. It worsened at the least likely moments. Doing the right things didn't alleviate it.

Being a hopeful person was not a blessing when I suffered from MMCD. I had too long to endure in a place where hope was counterproductive. I had to avoid the crushing disappointments.

What I had to concentrate on instead of hope, was endurance without knowledge or understanding, without monitoring or questioning.

It was months of blind endurance that brought my recovery.

13

WHAT HELP HINDERED

*"How can I explain it to you,
you will understand it less after
I have explained it?"*

Family Reunion **T. S. Eliot**

It may be difficult for a person to form an understanding of someone else's experience when it is fundamentally unlike anything that that person has experienced themselves. With skilled prompts and observations, bits and pieces of information can be gleaned about what it is like, enough for a diagnosis to be made. No more is needed.

My advice to people dealing with MMCD sufferers is to ask them as little as possible and avoid the question "Why?" at all costs.

The last person fit to answer the question "Why?" is someone in the throes of MMCD. Questions about causality (these are really difficult at the best of times) are liable to cause added distress to the patient.

When I expressed to the General Practitioner (G.P.) I saw that I was fearful without an immediate cause he would persist in trying to get me to talk about why I thought it was happening. I had no answer. Asking me "Why?" was like asking an amputee why he or she can feel discomfort from where a limb used to be. The mechanisms might not be clear to the sufferer. Furthermore knowing the reasons won't help the patient manage the discomfort. I can vouch for fear being a reality without any fear-inspiring occurrences to prompt it.

Once a diagnosis of MMCD has been confirmed it is important to focus on how to proceed to maximise the chances of survival, without getting side-tracked with the interesting subject of why it occurred or why the sensations arise once it has occurred.

In the early days of presenting with MMCD my G.P. asked me, in the few minutes at the end of the allotted consultation time, if I had had a happy childhood. I had more sense than to try to formulate an answer. If I had been compliant I would have been left high and dry with heightened emotions, unresolved questions and a deluge of thoughts, none of which I could afford in my condition. Even if, by some miracle, I had come up with a complete answer it would have been of no help in deciding what treatment I needed.

The possible reasons for a particular case of MMCD occurring are fascinating, not least to the sufferer. But when I was firmly steered away, by friends, from contemplating the causes of my illness I was undoubtedly helped significantly. The causes are too numerous, too deeply rooted and too multi-factorial to be of any immediate use. In an MMCD sufferer they are liable to overload an already over stretched capacity to think and feel.

Research done by those who are in a position to carry it out effectively is of great benefit to public health but MMCD sufferers are not equipped to undertake their own research while they are in the grips of the illness.

Being asked "Why do you think this has happened?" in the early days of MMCD was a bit like being asked by a mountain rescue team, before any help is offered, when you are hanging from a rope off a mountain in a snowstorm over a crevasse, when the frost bite is setting in and you are losing consciousness, "Why do you think you are in this condition?" and you feel like saying, amongst other things, "Could you help me before we discuss that?".

Another form of help that was unhelpful which occurred during both episodes of MMCD was people making false assumptions about my condition. I was not mentally agile enough to put them right. This would sometimes lead to them thinking they knew best about what would help me or what was possible.

Attempts to cheer me up were a problem. "You need cheering up! I'm coming to visit." It was taxing trying to convey that I wasn't suffering from a low mood and that meeting people made my condition worse. The pressure of not wanting to hurt people was intense and it could be difficult to convince people who had preconceived ideas. In these cases I think the word depression gave people the wrong idea. I had to say "No" a lot and try not to get involved in detailed explanations which were draining. This added to the problems I already had of saying "No" a lot to people, who were full of understanding of the condition and who I was most relaxed with, simply because it was a great strain to be in company with anyone.

I was told by some people that they themselves had nearly had a "*breakdown*" like me but they '*turned back*', so they knew what it was like for me. That didn't sound to me like my experience. My experience was more like walking through a field on a footpath where other people walked in complete safety. When I was in the middle of the field I got more and more scared without knowing why and then I saw a group of horses and I froze. Turning back wouldn't have got me out any quicker than continuing. Sensing my fear the horses went berserk and knocked me over.

Misunderstandings can be very alienating. If you jump to the conclusion that an MMCD sufferer is going through something you have experienced yourself, and you tell that person that you know you share common ground, it can be a real barrier for that person if it turns out not to be the case. I would recommend that it would be easier for an MMCD sufferer to have someone else's experience described to them and then to be left to draw his or her own conclusions as to whether there is any similarity or not. And that would only be appropriate if the sufferer asks.

People kindly try to reassure MMCD sufferers in many

different ways. Unfortunately, one thing it was not helpful to be told was that there is no longer a stigma attached to this illness (which I had no thoughts about at all and didn't mind about). It was rather like being singled out by your neighbour to be told that you won't encounter any discrimination based on your ethnic origins in this street (when you didn't expect you would). It was rather a strange experience.

One of the ways of helping I remember most vividly being unhelpful was the waiting to see the G.P. I had to wait for an indefinite period in a large open plan room where a large number of people, several of whom I knew, came and went. I was visible and had no conversation for them. In the early days I needed to get back home as soon as possible. The indefinite waiting was very difficult. My G.P. would walk past me to find the next patient without acknowledging me. Each time I saw him approaching I thought it would be my turn. My attention was on a helter skelter. I waited for an average of over 50 minutes for each of those early G.P. appointments, trying to remember to breathe regularly, being reassured by a friend, without whom I could not have stayed.

I was seeing the G.P. because I thought I had to in order to get a referral to a specialist and then to continue to get medication. It turned out that unbeknown to me I could have referred myself to the Community Mental Health Team, be assessed, have regular meetings and get medication without those gruelling visits (see later).

Waiting to see staff from the local Community Mental Health Team was a different prospect. There was no queuing. No-one broadcast my name (in the G.P.'s surgery my name was repeated loudly and also displayed in red on a large screen for the maximum number of people to see, as if it was on a timetable in an airport).

At the Community Mental Health team the scale was different, there was a small, usually empty waiting area not a large hall with many people coming and going. On the one occasion there that I wasn't seen within five minutes of arriving (which was because I had got the time wrong) I was told in advance that I would have to wait for fifteen minutes and I was offered a hot drink by someone who put me as much at my ease as was possible. In so doing, this person also gave me the reassurance that she knew what was going on and would oversee the situation. What I found very difficult was being unsure of what to expect while waiting and, at the Community Mental Health Team, unlike in the G.P. surgery, I didn't feel unsure about what was soon to happen.

The G.P. I saw would finish the meetings by unilaterally deciding that we must meet again and told me that I had to go out and make an appointment by queuing again at reception. Because of the state I was in, I tended to forget this between the G.P.'s door and the exit. This meant that when I got home I had another problem to solve.

The member of staff I saw at the Community Mental Health Team would make an offer of another appointment and we arranged the time and date between us face to face during the meeting, I didn't have to go elsewhere to do it.

The ratio of waiting time plus time taken to arrange appointments to the time spent meeting the G.P. was about 10:1. The equivalent with the Community Mental Health Team was much less than 1:10.

Apart from not being skilled at listening to or gaining information from someone who was in extremis, the G.P. was at a disadvantage from the start because I didn't disclose the extent of the problem. I didn't feel it was a good idea to tell someone who demonstrated little understanding of mental health problems (who would keep records that would be accessible to many others in the health professions from then onwards) that I was suicidal. The G.P. didn't know what was going on which was no fault of his own.

I found that the staff of the Community Mental Health Team could conceive that there was a lot going on that was not obvious and they got a feel of the hidden, by acute observations and skilled listening and not getting side-tracked by the surface appearances or answers to set questions. I also felt confidence in how the information I gave there would be interpreted and handled so I divulged a lot more.

14

WHAT HELP
TO ORGANISE
IN ADVANCE

I suggest that though there is no reason to believe you will suffer from MMCD in the future it is sensible to organise now how you would gain access to adequate services in the unlikely event of you needing them later, because the sort of treatment you find would critically affect whether you recover or not.

You may be able to get access to private services that would suit you.

At the time of going to press most people who get help for MMCD from the National Health Service do so by going first to their G.P. Some G.P.s will be skilled in getting the information required to diagnose MMCD ("Major Depression" or "Major Depressive Disorder" and some G.P.s won't. In some areas of the United Kingdom G.P.s will refer you to the local Community Mental Health Team and in some areas they won't. In some areas you can refer yourself to the Community Mental Health Team and in some areas you can't. The Community Mental Health Teams in some areas treat MMCD ("Major Depression, "Major Depressive

Disorder") and in some areas they will refer you back to the G.P.

If you are relying on the National Health Service then, unless you and your G.P. have a good rapport and mutual understanding and your G.P. is well informed about severe mental health problems, I think it is necessary to find (while you are well) another practitioner in advance of any future problems. Maybe you can find a G.P. in the same G.P.'s surgery who can help, or perhaps you will have to look at another G.P.'s surgery. Alternatively you may be able to refer yourself to the local Community Mental Health Team.

My hope is that, by asking, we will discover whether improvements need to be made in the provision of care. Do we have a workable system of self referral to Community Mental Health Teams? Do we need a specialised system in G.P.'s surgeries which offers contact from the start that is tailored to the needs of those suffering from MMCD? Do we need to know of the presence of at least one G.P. in each practice who has sufficient training in the problems associated with severe mental health problems to make adequate provision for specialist assessment and treatment?

If you do not find the services required I suggest you lobby for them.

What helped me was the full attention without interruption for up to *an hour or so* at a time, *of a person skilled in dealing with mental health problems* who had experience of treating similar conditions before, whose paid work was to help me, who remembered what had happened at our previous meetings, who I wasn't going to shock, who was not too stressed to listen effectively, from whom there was a reliable offer to continue such meetings and with whom there could be some confidentiality, some mutual respect and a rapport.

During these meetings I was given intelligent interpretations of what was happening to me as well as accurate assessments of what was to come. I was treated respectfully whilst not being asked to respond as if I had my full mental faculties. I was also assessed, diagnosed and, whilst trying medication, I was monitored until a successful dosage was reached. I was given a daytime phone number to call (which I used on about a dozen occasions) which allowed me to speak, on most occasions, within the hour, to the practitioner I had been meeting.

The treatment that helped me was given to me by the Community Mental Health Team which I struggled through the G.P. system to find. Some people find this sort of successful treatment with their G.P. Some people don't find it at all.

If you came to a standstill and had to take to your bed (you may find you revert to a state of infantile dependence for a period) the Community Mental Health Team may be able to offer a bed and care regarding your own immediate needs. If not, however, or if you would want to arrange another option, or if you have dependants to be taken care of, my advice is that you make investigations when you are well. You may want to agree with a group of friends that at any given time if one of you were in trouble you all know you would have adequate support from other members of the group.

Consider the sort of effects alcohol has on you (people vary a lot). I have decided in advance I would avoid alcohol.

Consider the pros and cons of medication for you. I once thought that a condition caused by psychological, behavioural and environmental factors as well as biochemical ones could only be healed by holistic means. I thought that a drug may be able to mask the problem but that the problem would remain to be solved at a later stage. But I have changed my mind since my experience of taking SSRIs in the last eighteen months. I know that they didn't just ease my symptoms. I am convinced that they helped me readjust my thought processes and the ways I feel emotions from a terrible state to a well functioning state.

You can find loads of information about research into medication and "Major Depression", if you are so inclined, in medical journals.

When I suffered from MMCD there were many periods when trying to concentrate my mind in conversation was deleterious and working with my awareness of my mental processes was counterproductive. I was simply not well enough. I am now wary of studies that do not distinguish carefully between different sorts of depression. Some have concluded that talking therapies are just as beneficial as medication. Imagine testing female contraceptive pills on everyone liable to procreate (without distinguishing between the different cases of men and women). The results would show that the pill was not as effective overall as rhythm methods. If, however, it is tested just on women, it is shown to be extremely effective. In the same way if you test SSRIs on all people with bad depressions you will not find out about their efficacy in treating people suffering from MMCD.

15

WHAT OTHER HELP HELPED

What also helped me when I had MMCD and when I was recovering was that I could contact, when I needed to, friends and family as well as health professionals who had the capacity to listen and keep an open mind. They knew that in order to find out how to communicate with me, it was effective to observe how I reacted and what I freely brought into the frame. They knew that answers I formulated literally to questions that required judgements would not be useful because we no longer shared the same terms of reference. They would know not to ask "So how are you?", a hideously huge and general question probing for a definitive answer. Friends would frame questions which required me to answer by my recounting what had happened rather than making a judgement. They would ask "What did you last have to eat?" and "When did you last sleep and for how long?" Or they just asked questions that were tangential, trivial and even easier to answer, such as, "Have you got warm bedclothes?" "Which room did you sleep in last, was it comfortable?" "Did you see the full moon?" and they listened intelligently to how I then spoke and what I chose to add.

As mentioned earlier, when I sent a text message or an e-mail I was not always very clear. "I'm ok" may have meant to me "My condition is worse than usual but I've got it under control."

My message saying that I was ok might get the reply "I hope you have a good day" which would normally be a lovely message but it left me wondering if I was completely beyond the pale, beyond reach or subhuman because all I could try for was minimising the pain of the day. Having a good day was tantalisingly out of reach, even a respite wouldn't last a whole day.

In contrast, the following message worked wonders for me: "Lovely to hear from you and to know that you are managing through the 'ups' and 'downs'. It doesn't make the 'downs' any nicer though does it?".

Another sort of useful message was "When you feel you can't go on for another minute change your immediate surroundings."

Because I was having contact with a G.P. who was not able to comprehend the situation it was reassuring and helpful to be in contact with some people who understood the long term picture.

It also helped when people responded to any specifics that I did communicate about, however trivial, so that I knew I was being heard.

If you are close to someone with MMCD it may help to think that he or she may long for a bed in a safe, quiet, empty, white room with no questions and no stimuli, being cared for like an animal is cared for by a vet rather than being asked to respond in some coherent way. The MMCD sufferer may be trying to get this sort of care from those nearest. Those nearest may be unable to fathom the selfishness of this person who can't be bothered, even after months of recovery, to function normally.

Sometimes there is nothing you can say to someone with MMCD that is right. MMCD will often be a great strain on marriages and friendships. I think that looking outside for help is more useful than looking for help within the relationship (for both people).

Having phone calls made for me and having my medication requested and collected for me by friends shielded me considerably.

Friends helped me enormously by accompanying me, reassuring me and acting as my eyes and ears on the few occasions I had to venture out when I was most ill. They reminded me of information that had been given to me when I had no recollection of it. On one occasion after a meeting at the Community Mental Health Team I thought the member of staff had given up on me. The friend who had been there helped me assess the evidence I had of this and I was enabled to see that the evidence to the contrary was, in fact, stronger.

I couldn't have managed without friends who, between them, offered me twenty four hour contact when I was at a standstill and who unobtrusively reiterated by text message and by e-mail that they could be contacled during the months when I chose not to see them and when I needed to be alone.

One friend of mine knew I used to enjoy walking. When I was recovering from MMCD he set up a time each week when he would leave me a message to see if I would come out for a stroll that we could turn back from at any stage if I wanted. He insisted that if I declined the offer of meeting he wouldn't mind and I did decline about five weeks out of six. The way he offered these walks was valuable. It was important for me at that stage that I wasn't attempting activities I would fail at and I didn't want to cause a friend constant disappointment, so his guarantee that he didn't mind if I declined his offers time after time, and at the last minute too, was crucial to me.

My friends and family consistently showed this sort of consideration.

It was very heartening that after a year of minimal physical movement and a great deal of lying down, my muscles hadn't atrophied. After the illness my body functioned quite well. It may not have been useful at the time for me to reflect on this but it may be useful to onlookers to be reassured how tenaciously the body holds on to life.

I took to reminding myself, when I was very incapacitated, that I was the same person as I was when I was having a respite. As yet, the person who at times felt normal had not been destroyed by this condition however bad it felt in the moment.

After many months I could start to believe that the illness would end one day, however many times I would have bad experiences or recurrences of the lurching horrors before that. For the first time the overall course of the illness was towards recovery, bumpy and gradual though the improvement was. The periods when I felt normal were progressively lengthening and occurring more frequently. At last hope became useful. I could safely now start to believe what people had been telling me : it would end, we just didn't know when.

"It will end, we just don't know when". I recited it like a mantra.

I started to believe that however long it would stretch out ahead of me it really would end at some future point.

So every minute, every second that I got through was one minute or one second off the total time span of the illness.

POSTSCRIPT

My experiences are not the same as other people's experiences and these personal accounts cannot inform about others' cases. But I hope other people who have experienced MMCD will use these accounts as a stepping stone to describe their own experiences and improve the common knowledge of this condition so that sufferers no longer have to be set back by counterproductive sessions with G.P.'s and struggles with people who have no conception of what is going on.

My first episode of MMCD left me considerably mentally weaker for a decade than I had been before. My second episode of MMCD was more horrific than the first and I was closer to suicide than I had been in the first episode, but it didn't leave me as weak once I had recovered.

If I had not been helped by the SSRI I was prescribed during my second episode of MMCD I don't think I could have hung on to try another. Who can say? If I had not been so determined to eat or if I had not been able to keep food down, I don't think I would have recovered. If I had been living with someone in the second episode of MMCD (as I had been during my first episode) I don't know how I could have recovered as well. The difficulties of trying to minimise my effect on a partner took its toll on me during my first episode.

In my second episode of MMCD I had a chaotic sleep routine with no difference between day and night for months, articles of clothing were dropped and not touched for days, I was erratic and irrational and wanted to be left completely alone. I listened to audio tapes ceaselessly, I turned the phone and answer phone off for twelve months and couldn't explain what was going on. Not conducive to good marital relations.

My first episode of MMCD was more disorientating to me than my second episode was and I had a negative outlook: the world seemed to have gone wrong. In the second episode (except at the beginning) I had quite an optimistic view of the world. The world seemed ok, but I had gone wrong.

During both episodes I had to fight the idea that occurred to me that I was being punished. I thought I might be being punished for having had too good a life. I know that some MMCD sufferers feel they are being punished because they are bad. If I had been fixed on that idea, I think my recovery would have been harder.

A lot of people turn to alcohol which usually hinders recovery from MMCD and I may well have done that if I didn't have such an abiding memory of how my symptoms worsened the day after a drink, however much a drink helped me at the time. Because of that I was scared of drinking and kept teetotal for the entire second episode.

People with MMCD often worsen their conditions by turning to erratic or excessive doses of other mind-altering substances.

I am left with the knowledge that it could have been worse for me and that other people have it worse.

I survived and I get lots of pats on the back for that but some other people try just as hard, have it worse and don't survive.